Healing with the AIP Diet

Simple Recipes and Strategies to Restore Balance
and Fight Inflammation with AIP

J. Waller

Introduction

Describe the AIP Diet.

Many people struggle with inexplicable symptoms and health issues in a society when the quick speed of life sometimes overcomes our well-being. Among these, autoimmune illnesses are proliferating and affecting millions of lives. The Autoimmune Protocol (AIP) Diet is a transforming method of healing that transcends only symptom management if you have been looking for a solution offering more than just temporary comfort.

For people with autoimmune diseases especially, the AIP Diet is not only another food trend; it's a whole treatment program meant to bring the body back into equilibrium. Fundamentally, the AIP Diet emphasizes on cutting foods and drugs that could aggravate inflammation while also supporting complete meals high in nutrients that heal and nourish. This seeks to reset your immune system and intestinal health, therefore lowering the inflammation driving autoimmune illnesses.

The knowledge that many chronic diseases result from a mix of environmental elements including nutrition and genetic inclination drives the Autoimmune Protocol. The AIP Diet gently eliminates possibly dangerous foods such grains, dairy, legumes, nightshade vegetables, and processed sweets and substitutes nourishing foods including vegetables, fruits, lean meats, and healthy fats. This rigorous approach not only benefits in symptom management but also fosters a stronger awareness of how the foods we consume effect our general well-being.

Explanation of the Autoimmune Protocol

The AIP Diet is divided in two phases: elimination and reintroduction. During the elimination phase, you'll remove all probable inflammatory items from your diet for a predetermined duration, usually about 30 to 90 days. This is a key step, allowing your body the time it needs to heal and recover from the chronic inflammation that may have been aggravated by food choices.

After the elimination phase, the reintroduction phase begins. This is where the magic truly happens. You'll gradually reintroduce particular foods back into your diet, one at a time, while carefully monitoring your body's response. This technique not only helps discover particular food triggers but also enables you to take care of your health by learning how various meals affect your individual body.

The AIP Diet isn't only about what you avoid; it's also about what you add. It's an opportunity to explore a wide selection of nutrient-rich foods, fostering creativity and discovery in the kitchen. From colorful vegetable stir-fries to savory, slow-cooked meats, the AIP Diet celebrates the joy of cooking and eating healthily, ensuring that you never feel restricted.

Overview of Its Origins and Purpose

The origins of the AIP Diet may be traced back to the Paleo diet, which stresses full, unprocessed foods while excluding grains, dairy, and legumes. The AIP Diet develops upon this basis, adapting it specifically for patients with autoimmune illnesses. Developed by researchers, healthcare practitioners, and individuals with firsthand experience in managing autoimmune disorders, the AIP nutrition is a result of years of research into the link between nutrition, inflammation, and autoimmune responses.

The major goal of the AIP Diet is to create a structured framework for healing. By emphasizing on nutrient-dense foods and eliminating those that may trigger inflammation, the AIP Diet tries to:

Reduce Inflammation: Chronic inflammation is typically at the basis of autoimmune disorders. The AIP Diet provides a clear approach for lowering this inflammation through dietary adjustments.

Heal the Gut: A healthy gut is necessary for effective immunological function. The AIP Diet emphasizes foods that support gut health, creating a diverse and balanced microbiota.

Empower Individuals: The AIP Diet supports personal empowerment through food choices. By learning to listen to your body and understand how it reacts to certain foods, you can take charge of your health.

Support Overall Wellness: Beyond only addressing autoimmune symptoms, the AIP Diet fosters a holistic approach to health, stressing physical, emotional, and mental well-being.

Why Focus on Healing and Inflammation?

For many, the journey toward healing typically begins with the recognition that standard methods to health may not always be sufficient. While drugs might provide relief, they typically come with a plethora of adverse effects and may not address the underlying reasons of autoimmune disorders. This is where the AIP Diet excels, delivering a proactive and empowered approach to health.

Focusing on healing and inflammation is vital since inflammation is a key player in many chronic diseases, particularly autoimmune ones.

When the body is in a permanent state of inflammation, it can lead to a cascade of negative health impacts, aggravating symptoms and contributing to disease development. By managing inflammation through dietary adjustments, individuals can create a more favorable internal environment that promotes recovery.

The relevance of inflammation cannot be emphasized. It serves as the body's normal response to injury or infection, but when it becomes chronic, it can lead to major health concerns. For patients with autoimmune illnesses, this persistent inflammation can cause a number of symptoms, including fatigue, discomfort, digestive difficulties, and cognitive dysfunction.

By embracing the AIP Diet, you are taking a proactive stand in your health quest. Rather than passively managing symptoms, you are actively attempting to uncover and eliminate the fundamental causes of your inflammation. This transformation in mindset—from reactive to proactive—can be very empowering, leading to substantial changes in your quality of life.

__Personal Stories & Testimonials__

The strength of the AIP Diet lies not only in its scientific basis but also in the many human stories of transformation and healing. Individuals from many walks of life have embraced the AIP Diet and enjoyed incredible benefits, reclaiming their health and well-being.

One inspiring story comes from Sarah, a 34-year-old mother of two who fought with rheumatoid arthritis for over a decade. After years of relying on pain drugs with minimal success, Sarah discovered upon the AIP Diet. Skeptical but hopeful, she committed to the elimination phase, hoping to give her body a chance to heal. Within weeks, she noted a considerable reduction in joint discomfort and weariness. The lively energy she had thought was lost began to resurface, allowing her to engage fully with her children. Today, Sarah continues to flourish on the AIP Diet, and her experience has encouraged many others in her community to investigate the healing potential of dietary changes.

Similarly, John, a 45-year-old veteran, experienced painful symptoms of multiple sclerosis for years. Despite trying several treatments, he felt stuck in his own body. After discovering the AIP Diet through an online support group, John was intrigued by the potential of taking control of his health. He dived into the elimination phase, focusing on nutritious foods and making lifestyle adjustments. To his amazement, John's symptoms began to lessen, and he discovered newfound hope and vigor. Today, he actively shares his journey with others, urging them to discover the healing potential of the AIP Diet.

These personal stories show a growing community of individuals who have embraced the AIP Diet not just as a temporary remedy but as a lifelong commitment to health and fitness. They reflect the spirit of perseverance and persistence, suggesting that recovery is achievable through dietary choices and lifestyle modifications.

As you embark on your journey through Healing with the AIP Diet, I ask you to approach it with an open mind and a readiness to explore new possibilities. The route to healing may not always be easy, but it is surely rewarding. You are not alone in your journey; numerous others have taken the same path and emerged stronger, healthier, and more vibrant.

Through this book, you will find not just recipes and practical ideas but also a sense of community and support. Together, we will negotiate the intricacies of the AIP Diet, celebrating each step toward health and balance. Your adventure begins today, and I am delighted to take you through the transforming potential of the Autoimmune Protocol.

In the chapters that follow, you will discover simple, tasty recipes, meal planning suggestions, and personal anecdotes that will motivate you to embrace the AIP Diet fully. Let's go on this road toward healing together, one wholesome meal at a time.

Chapter 1: Understanding Inflammation and Autoimmunity

What is Inflammation?

Inflammation is a complex biological response of the body's immune system to damaging stimuli, such as bacteria, damaged cells, or irritants. It is a crucial aspect of the body's healing process, serving as a defense mechanism that helps to fight off infections and initiate recovery. However, not all inflammation is good, and understanding the different types of inflammation is vital for grasping how it links to autoimmune illnesses.

Types of Inflammation: Acute vs. Chronic

Inflammation can be categorized into two major types: acute and chronic.

Acute Inflammation

Acute inflammation is the body's first response to damage or infection. It is a short-term process that normally lasts from a few hours to a few days. This type of inflammation is marked by five traditional signs: redness, heat, swelling, pain, and loss of function. When you stub your toe or acquire a sore throat, these symptoms are signs of acute inflammation at work.

The process of acute inflammation involves multiple steps:

Recognition of Harmful Stimuli: When tissues are wounded or infected, the body's immune cells recognize the threat.

Vasodilation: Blood vessels enlarge, boosting blood flow to the affected area. This is what creates the redness and heat.

Increased Permeability: Blood arteries become more permeable, allowing vital immune cells, proteins, and nutrients to reach the site of injury or infection.

Immune Cell Recruitment: White blood cells, particularly neutrophils, move to the site of inflammation to attack pathogens and clear away debris.

Acute inflammation is often protective and disappears once the underlying cause is treated. However, if the triggering element persists, acute inflammation can evolve into chronic inflammation.

__Chronic Inflammation__

Chronic inflammation, on the other hand, is a protracted inflammatory response that can linger for months or even years. It often emerges when the body fails to eradicate the initial cause of inflammation or when the immune system mistakenly assaults healthy tissues, as seen in autoimmune illnesses. Unlike acute inflammation, chronic inflammation is not usually accompanied by the classic indications of redness or swelling, making it insidious and often difficult to detect.

Chronic inflammation can lead to a wide array of health concerns, including:

Autoimmune Diseases: Conditions when the immune system assaults the body's own tissues.

Cardiovascular Diseases: Chronic inflammation can damage blood arteries and contribute to heart disease.

Metabolic Disorders: Conditions like obesity and type 2 diabetes are connected with chronic inflammation.

The body's failure to manage inflammation can lead to a vicious cycle, where inflammation perpetuates itself, causing tissue damage and malfunction.

Role of Inflammation in the Body

Inflammation has several key roles in preserving health:

Defense Against illnesses: By targeting pathogens and infected cells, inflammation helps the body ward against illnesses.

Tissue Repair: Inflammation initiates the healing process, allowing for tissue regeneration and repair after injury.

Regulation of Immune Responses: Inflammation helps regulate the immune response, ensuring that the body responds correctly to threats without overreacting.

While inflammation is necessary for health, its persistence can have the opposite effect, leading to chronic illnesses. This duality underlines the significance of establishing balance within the body and identifying the signals that inflammation may have crossed the line from helpful to harmful.

Autoimmune Diseases Explained

Autoimmune illnesses constitute a key consequence of chronic inflammation, characterized by the immune system's mistaken attack on the body's own cells and tissues. This misguided response can lead to many health complications, as the immune system fails to distinguish between hazardous invaders and healthy cells.

Common Autoimmune Diseases and Their Symptoms

There are around 80 recognized autoimmune illnesses, each with its distinct set of symptoms and manifestations. Some of the most common include:

Rheumatoid Arthritis (RA):

Symptoms: Joint discomfort, stiffness, edema, weariness, and sometimes fever.

effect: RA primarily affects the joints but can also effect organs and systems throughout the body.

Lupus (Systemic Lupus Erythematosus):

Symptoms: Fatigue, joint pain, skin rashes, and fever, with phases of exacerbation and remission.

Impact: Lupus can affect several organs, including the heart, kidneys, and brain.

Multiple Sclerosis (MS):

Symptoms: Numbness, weakness, eyesight issues, and cognitive changes.

Impact: MS begins when the immune system destroys the protective covering of nerves, resulting to communication difficulties between the brain and the body.

Hashimoto's Thyroiditis:

Symptoms: Fatigue, weight gain, cold intolerance, and sadness.

Impact: This disorder results in an underactive thyroid (hypothyroidism) because to the immune system destroying thyroid tissue.

Type 1 Diabetes:

Symptoms: Increased thirst, frequent urination, weariness, and impaired vision.

Impact: In Type 1 diabetes, the immune system destroys insulin-producing cells in the pancreas, leading to high blood sugar levels.

Celiac Disease:

Symptoms: Digestive difficulties, tiredness, and skin rashes.

Impact: This autoimmune illness is produced by the ingestion of gluten, leading to inflammation in the intestines.

While these disorders differ in their precise symptoms and affected locations, they share a common underlying theme: chronic inflammation plays a crucial role in their genesis and progression.

How Inflammation Affects Autoimmune Conditions

The link between inflammation and autoimmune disorders is deep and multifaceted. In autoimmune disorders, the immune system wrongly perceives the body's own cells as foreign invaders, triggering an inflammatory reaction. This can lead to a cycle of harm and repair that becomes self-perpetuating, ultimately damaging the individual's health.

Tissue Damage:

Inflammation can cause severe damage to tissues and organs, leading to discomfort, malfunction, and disability. For example, in rheumatoid arthritis, the immune system targets the synovial tissue in the joints, resulting in inflammation and joint damage.

Increased Immune Activation:

Chronic inflammation can sustain immune system activation, causing the body to remain in a permanent state of alert. This heightened immune response might result in the destruction of healthy tissues and worsen autoimmune symptoms.

Gut Health:

The health of the gut plays a significant role in inflammation and autoimmune disorders. An imbalanced gut microbiome, defined by an abundance of dangerous bacteria and a dearth of healthy ones, can contribute to systemic inflammation. The gut lining can become permeable (commonly referred to as "leaky gut"), allowing toxins and undigested food particles to enter the bloodstream and further stimulate the immune system.

Environmental Triggers:

Various environmental factors, such as nutrition, stress, infections, and pollutants, can alter inflammation levels and provoke autoimmune reactions. For instance, certain foods may elicit an immunological response in vulnerable individuals, while stress can lead to hormonal changes that increase inflammation.

Autoantibodies:

In many autoimmune illnesses, the immune system creates autoantibodies—antibodies that wrongly target and attack the body's own tissues. This can lead to chronic inflammation and more tissue damage, creating a vicious cycle.

The Importance of Understanding Inflammation and Autoimmunity

Understanding the relationship between inflammation and autoimmune disorders is crucial for establishing successful treatment solutions. Recognizing the indicators of chronic inflammation and addressing its fundamental causes through dietary and lifestyle changes can empower individuals to take charge of their health.

The Autoimmune Protocol (AIP) Diet acts as a valuable aid in this quest. By focusing on anti-inflammatory foods and removing potential triggers, the AIP Diet attempts to reduce inflammation, support gut health, and promote overall well-being.

As we go deeper into the chapters ahead, we will discuss the practical components of the AIP Diet, including meal planning, delectable recipes, and techniques to overcome the hurdles of this transforming dietary strategy. Armed with knowledge and practical tools, you can take charge of your health and go on a journey of healing and rejuvenation.

In this chapter, we have created the framework for understanding the crucial roles that inflammation and autoimmunity play in our health. By recognizing the indicators of inflammation and how it can emerge in autoimmune disorders, we set the stage for investigating practical techniques to restore balance within the body.

The journey toward healing is a path of discovery, and with each step, you will gain insights into how your body functions and what it needs to thrive. Armed with the knowledge of inflammation and autoimmune, you are now prepared to embrace the transforming potential of the AIP Diet, taking a huge step toward regaining your health and well-being.

Chapter 2: The Science Behind AIP

How AIP Works

The Autoimmune Protocol (AIP) Diet is more than simply a restrictive diet plan; it is a complete approach to healing that targets the fundamental causes of autoimmune diseases. At its foundation, AIP is designed to identify and remove items that can provoke inflammation while simultaneously providing the body with therapeutic nutrients. To appreciate how AIP works, we must delve into its mechanisms of action and understand the important role of gut health in autoimmune illnesses.

Mechanisms of Action: Removing Inflammatory Triggers

The AIP Diet operates on the concept that some foods might induce inflammation and worsen autoimmune symptoms. By systematically eliminating these inflammatory triggers, AIP allows the body to reset, repair, and reestablish balance. Here's how it works:

Elimination of Potential Triggers

The AIP Diet removes a wide variety of foods believed to contribute to inflammation and autoimmune. These include:

Grains: Wheat, rice, and corn can elicit immunological responses in some individuals.

Legumes: Beans and lentils can be irritating for people with sensitivity.

Dairy: Dairy products can worsen inflammation and digestive difficulties.

Processed Foods: Packaged foods often contain chemicals, preservatives, and harmful fats that can induce inflammation.

Nightshade Vegetables: Tomatoes, peppers, and eggplants might induce flare-ups in certain people.

Sugar: High sugar intake is associated to increased inflammation and chronic illnesses.

Alcohol: Alcohol can disturb gut health and cause inflammation.

By removing certain foods from the diet, individuals can decrease their exposure to possible triggers and give their immune systems a chance to calm down.

Nutrient-Dense Foods for Healing

AIP advocates the consumption of nutrient-dense foods that assist the body's healing processes. This includes:

Vegetables: Leafy greens, cruciferous vegetables, and other colorful veggies contain critical vitamins, minerals, and antioxidants.

Fruits: Low-sugar fruits, such as berries and apples, are rich in antioxidants that help battle oxidative stress.

Healthy Fats: Avocado, olive oil, and coconut oil provide anti-inflammatory effects and necessary fatty acids.

Quality Proteins: Grass-fed meats, wild-caught fish, and pasture-raised poultry contain critical nutrients and assist support muscle and tissue repair.

Bone Broth: Packed in collagen and amino acids, bone broth improves digestive healing and helps joint health.

The combination of limiting inflammatory meals and embracing nutrient-dense options promotes an atmosphere conducive to recovery.

Gradual Reintroduction of Foods

After a period of elimination (typically 30-90 days), individuals can begin to reintroduce removed foods one at a time. This approach helps detect specific food sensitivities and enables individuals to customize their diets to their unique needs. By studying how the body responds to each item, individuals can make informed selections about what to include in their long-term eating habits.

Immune System Regulation

The AIP Diet may also alter the immune system's functioning. By lowering inflammation and supporting gut healing, the immune system can begin to control itself more effectively. This can lead to a decrease in the generation of autoantibodies—proteins that wrongly attack the body's own tissues. Over time, this management can help reduce autoimmune symptoms and enhance general health.

Role of Gut Health in Autoimmune Diseases

The stomach plays a key function in the immune system and overall health. In fact, nearly 70% of the immune system lies in the gut. Understanding the relationship between gut health and autoimmunity is key for appreciating the science underpinning AIP.

The Gut Barrier

The gut lining functions as a protective barrier that limits what enters the bloodstream. When the gut is healthy, it permits important nutrients to pass while inhibiting harmful things. However, a damaged gut lining (commonly referred to as "leaky gut") can contribute to increased intestinal permeability. This disorder permits toxins, undigested food particles, and microorganisms to enter the circulation, generating an immunological response that can contribute to inflammation and autoimmune.

The Microbiome

The gut microbiome—the population of billions of bacteria and other microorganisms living in the digestive tract—plays a critical role in maintaining gut health and supporting immune function. A diversified and balanced microbiota can help manage inflammation and protect against autoimmune diseases. Conversely, an imbalance in gut flora (dysbiosis) has been related to greater inflammation and a higher risk of autoimmune disorders.

Diet's Impact on Gut Health

The foods we eat directly influence the composition and diversity of the gut microbiome. A diet rich in fiber, fruits, vegetables, and fermented foods can maintain a healthy microbiome, while a diet high in sugar, processed foods, and harmful fats can promote dysbiosis. The AIP Diet emphasizes foods that nourish the gut and support a balanced microbiota, ultimately creating a healthier immune response.

Inflammation and Gut Health

Chronic inflammation can harm the gut lining and change the microbiome, leading to a vicious cycle. By following the AIP Diet and reducing inflammation, individuals can support gut healing and restore balance to their microbiota, contributing to increased immune function and overall health.

Benefits of the AIP Diet

The AIP Diet offers a wide array of benefits that extend beyond simply lowering inflammation and managing inflammatory symptoms. While many people initially choose AIP for its anti-inflammatory properties, the good outcomes can span physical, emotional, and mental health advantages.

Physical, Emotional, and Mental Health Improvements

Physical Health Improvements

Many individuals claim major physical changes after adopting the AIP Diet, including:

Reduced Inflammation: One of the most immediate effects of AIP is a reduction in inflammation-related symptoms, such as joint pain, fatigue, and skin concerns. By avoiding inflammatory causes and supporting the body with healthy nutrients, individuals can enjoy relief from chronic discomfort.

Improved Digestion: The focus on gut health and nutrient-dense diets can lead to better digestion and nutrition absorption. Many people report that their digestive difficulties, such as bloating and gas, improve considerably on the AIP Diet.

Enhanced Energy Levels: With lower inflammation and enhanced nutritional absorption, many individuals report higher energy levels and a stronger sense of vitality. The AIP Diet encourages regulated blood sugar levels, which can also contribute to prolonged energy throughout the day.

Emotional Health Improvements

The connection between food and mental health is well-established. As individuals reduce inflammation and enhance their physical health, they often feel favorable changes in their emotional well-being:

Reduced Anxiety and Depression: Many persons with autoimmune disorders report heightened levels of anxiety and depression. By reducing physical symptoms and increasing general health, the AIP Diet can contribute to a more positive emotional state.

Better Mood Stability: A nutrient-rich diet can significantly influence neurotransmitter production and brain function. Improved gut health may also enhance the production of serotonin, a neurotransmitter associated with mood control, leading to greater emotional stability.

Mental Health Improvements

The AIP Diet may also boost cognitive function and mental clarity. Some benefits include:

Improved Focus and Concentration: Many people find that as they embrace the AIP Diet, their mental clarity increases. This can be particularly crucial for those experiencing "brain fog" as a consequence of their inflammatory disorder.

Enhanced Memory: A diet rich in antioxidants, healthy fats, and vitamins can support brain health and increase memory performance. The AIP Diet emphasizes nutrients that nourish the brain, potentially contributing to cognitive benefits.

Long-term vs. Short-term Benefits

While the AIP Diet delivers numerous immediate benefits, it is vital to acknowledge the possible long-term advantages of this dietary approach as well.

Short-term Benefits

Symptom Relief: Many persons see a reduction in autoimmune symptoms within weeks of adopting the AIP Diet. This can include decreased pain, improved digestion, and enhanced energy levels.

Increased Awareness: The process of eliminating and reintroducing foods promotes a greater understanding of one's body and its particular demands. This enhanced awareness can empower individuals to make informed food choices in the future.

Long-term Benefits

Sustained Health Improvements: Many people find that the favorable effects of the AIP Diet extend beyond the first elimination phase. Continued adherence to a modified AIP approach can lead to long-term gains in overall health, including lower risk of chronic diseases.

Preventing Autoimmune Flare-ups: By identifying and avoiding certain triggers, individuals can limit the risk of autoimmune flare-ups and keep better control over their health.

Lifestyle improvements: Embracing the AIP Diet frequently leads to lasting improvements in food habits and lifestyle choices. Many individuals gain a stronger appreciation for complete, nutrient-dense foods, leading to increased overall health and well-being.

__*Empowerment and Community*__

Engaging in the AIP community can give extra long-term benefits. Support from others on a similar journey can develop a sense of connection and empowerment, helping individuals feel less alienated in their challenges with autoimmunity. Sharing experiences, recipes, and advice can establish a strong support network that supports continuous achievement.

The research underlying the Autoimmune Protocol Diet is anchored in the study of inflammation, gut health, and the immune system. By avoiding inflammatory triggers and embracing nutrient-dense diets, individuals can enjoy tremendous physical, emotional, and mental health changes. The AIP Diet not only tackles the immediate symptoms of autoimmune disorders but also promotes long-term well-being and a restored sense of empowerment.

Chapter 3: Getting Started with AIP

Embarking on a path toward healing with the Autoimmune Protocol (AIP) Diet can feel both exhilarating and intimidating. The potential of lowering inflammation, recovering your health, and eventually increasing your quality of life is immensely inspiring. However, adjusting to this new way of eating involves significant planning and preparation. This chapter will walk you through the early steps to make the transition smoother, create a friendly kitchen atmosphere, and equip you with an important shopping list to get you started.

Initial Steps to Transition

Transitioning to the AIP Diet is not only about altering what you eat; it is a holistic approach that includes analyzing your current behaviors and creating an environment that encourages healing.

Assessment of Current Diet and Habits

Before jumping headfirst into the AIP Diet, it's necessary to take a step back and analyze your existing eating patterns and lifestyle. This assessment will serve as the foundation for your move and help you find areas for improvement.

Keep a Food Diary

Start by keeping a food journal for at least a week. Document everything you eat and drink, along with any symptoms you feel. Pay attention to how different foods affect your mood, energy levels, digestion, and autoimmune symptoms. This record will help you detect patterns and potential triggers that may need to be eliminated in your AIP journey.

___Identify Common Triggers___

As you evaluate your food diary, search for foods or substances that seem to coincide with flare-ups or bad symptoms. Common culprits in autoimmune diseases include gluten, dairy, sugar, and processed foods. Understanding your body's unique sensitivities to different foods will allow you to make informed decisions as you move to AIP.

___Set Clear Goals___

Establish your personal goals for adopting the AIP Diet. Do you wish to reduce inflammation, enhance digestion, or raise energy levels? Setting precise, achievable goals will keep you motivated and focused on your trip. Remember to write these goals down; keeping them visible will act as a reminder of why you picked this path.

Educate Yourself

Knowledge is power. Take time to read books, articles, and information concerning the AIP Diet and autoimmune disorders. Familiarizing yourself with the science behind the diet will improve your comprehension and empower you with confidence as you embark on this path.

Creating a Supportive Environment (Kitchen Tips)

A supportive atmosphere is crucial for effectively shifting to the AIP Diet. Your kitchen should be a haven of healing and nourishment, where nutritious foods are conveniently accessible. Here are some recommendations for constructing an AIP-friendly kitchen:

Declutter Your Pantry

Start by cleaning up your pantry and refrigerator. Remove any foods that are not AIP-compliant, including as grains, legumes, dairy, processed snacks, and refined sugars. Be honest with yourself about what you need to let go of. This decluttering exercise can be cathartic and will make it easier to resist temptation when you're faced with desires.

Organize AIP-Friendly Staples

Once your kitchen is decluttered, stock it with AIP-friendly basics. Organize these foods in a way that makes them conveniently accessible. This could include constructing a special shelf for AIP ingredients or using clear containers to store snacks and essentials. Having your kitchen set up for success will make meal planning and cooking more fun.

Meal Prep

Consider setting out a few hours each week for meal prep. Preparing AIP-compliant meals in advance will save you time during hectic weekdays and guarantee that you always have nutritious options on hand. Cook huge batches of soup, stews, or roasted veggies, and store them in portioned containers for convenient access.

Invest in Kitchen Tools

Equip your kitchen with crucial tools that will make cooking AIP-friendly meals easier. Consider investing in:

High-quality knives: A nice knife set will make chopping vegetables and preparing dishes more efficient.

Slow cooker or Instant Pot: These gadgets are wonderful for making soups, stews, and meats with minimal effort.

Blender or food processor: Great for creating smoothies, sauces, and nut butters.

Quality cookware: Invest in non-toxic pots and pans that are free from dangerous chemicals.

Create a Calm Cooking Space

Cooking can be a therapeutic pastime. Take time to establish a quiet and inviting cooking atmosphere in your kitchen. Play relaxing music, light candles, or add plants to improve the environment. When you feel good in your kitchen space, you're more likely to enjoy meal prep and experimentation.

Shopping List Essentials

With your kitchen prepared, it's time to tackle your shopping list. Knowing what to buy helps expedite your grocery excursions and guarantee that you have plenty of AIP-friendly options at home.

AIP-Friendly Foods and Ingredients

Here's a thorough shopping list to get you started on your AIP journey:

Fruits and Vegetables

Leafy greens (spinach, kale, collard greens)

Cruciferous vegetables (broccoli, cauliflower, Brussels sprouts)

Root veggies (sweet potatoes, carrots, beets)

Squash (zucchini, butternut squash, spaghetti squash)

Low-sugar fruits (berries, apples, pears, avocados)

Bananas with coconuts for snacks and desserts

Quality Proteins

Grass-fed beef, lamb, or bison

Pasture-raised chicken or turkey

Wild-caught fish (salmon, mackerel, sardines)

Organ meats (liver, heart, etc. for their nutritious density)

Eggs (if tolerated; can be reintroduced after the elimination phase)

Healthy Fats

Olive oil and avocado oil for cooking

Coconut oil for baking and sautéing

Avocados for snacks and salads

Nut and seed butters (such as sunflower seed butter)

Herbs & Spices

Fresh herbs (parsley, basil, cilantro)

Dried herbs and spices (turmeric, ginger, cinnamon)

Sea salt and Himalayan pink salt

Bone Broth and Fermented Foods

Homemade or store-bought bone broth for soups and healing

AIP-compliant fermented foods (like sauerkraut or kombucha) for gut health

Coconut Products

Canned coconut milk for creamy meals

Unsweetened shredded coconut for baking or snacks

Coconut flour for baking and cooking

Other AIP-Friendly Items

AIP-compliant foods (such as veggie chips or plantain chips)

Cacao powder for chocolate recipes

Honey or maple syrup as natural sweeteners (in moderation)

Avoiding Common Triggers

As you shop for AIP-friendly foods, it's crucial to be aware of frequent triggers to avoid. Here's a list of goods you should steer clear of:

Grains

Wheat, barley, rye, oats, and all gluten-containing grains

Rice, corn, and pseudo-grains like quinoa or buckwheat

Legumes

Beans, lentils, chickpeas, and peanuts

Dairy

Milk, cheese, yogurt, and all dairy products

Nightshade Vegetables

Tomatoes, potatoes, eggplants, peppers, and spices produced from them (like paprika)

Processed Foods

Anything containing chemicals, preservatives, and unhealthy fats

Sugar, including refined sugars, syrups, and sweetened beverages

Alcohol

All alcoholic beverages, as they might irritate the gut and increase inflammation

Refined Oils

Canola oil, soybean oil, and other processed vegetable oils that can contribute to inflammation

Getting started with the AIP Diet is a powerful and transforming journey. By examining your present habits, creating a supportive kitchen environment, and equipping yourself with a necessary shopping list, you're setting the stage for healing and regeneration. Remember, this journey is not about deprivation; it's about supporting your body with nutritious, therapeutic meals.

As you move forward, approach this process with an open mind and a willingness to learn. Your body is unique, and the AIP Diet can help you identify the foods that work best for you. In the next chapter, we will explore tasty AIP-friendly recipes that make this healing path not only nutritious but also enjoyable. Your voyage into the world of healing with the AIP Diet is just begun!

Chapter 4: Meal Planning and Preparation

Embarking on the Autoimmune Protocol (AIP) Diet is a transforming journey toward healing and restoring balance to your body. One of the most effective ways to ensure your success on this route is through diligent meal planning and preparation. By organizing your meals ahead of time, you may lessen the burden of everyday cooking, assure compliance with AIP rules, and ultimately cultivate a more joyful and sustainable lifestyle. In this chapter, we'll look into how to establish a weekly meal plan, investigate successful batch cooking procedures, and address fundamental cooking techniques that will increase your culinary experience while maintaining the nutrients in your food.

How to Create a Weekly Meal Plan

Creating a weekly meal plan is a vital step in ensuring that you stay on track with your AIP Diet. A well-structured meal plan allows you to keep diversity in your diet, limit food waste, and streamline your grocery shopping.

Sample Meal Planning Templates

Here are a couple templates to help you get started with your weekly food planning:

Basic Weekly Meal Plan Template

A simple layout can be incredibly effective. Create a chart with the days of the week across the top and meal slots for breakfast, lunch, dinner, and snacks in the columns below. For example:

Day Breakfast Lunch Dinner Snacks

Monday AIP Smoothie Chicken Salad Beef Stew Carrot Sticks

Tuesday Scrambled Eggs Vegetable Stir-Fry Baked Salmon Apple Slices

Wednesday Sweet Potato Hash Turkey Lettuce Wraps Zucchini Noodles Coconut Yogurt

Thursday Chia Seed Pudding Quinoa Bowl Stuffed Bell Peppers Dried Mango

Friday Green Smoothie AIP Tacos Grilled Chicken Plantain Chips

Saturday Banana Pancakes Soup Roasted Vegetables Cucumber Slices

Sunday Omelette Salad Spaghetti Squash Trail Mix

Detailed Weekly Meal Planner

This template can include specific recipes or components for each meal. You can customize the meal planning template to include additional areas for grocery lists or notes on what to prep in advance.

Day Breakfast Lunch Dinner Snacks Prep Notes

Monday AIP Smoothie with Spinach Chicken Salad with Olive Oil Beef Stew with Carrots and Peas Carrot Sticks with Guacamole Soak beans for stew overnight

Tuesday Scrambled Eggs with Herbs Vegetable Stir-Fry with Coconut Oil Baked Salmon with Asparagus Apple Slices with Cinnamon Chop veggies for stir-fry

Wednesday Sweet Potato Hash with Avocado Turkey Lettuce Wraps Zucchini Noodles with Meat Sauce Coconut Yogurt with Berries Cook additional turkey for wraps

Thursday Chia Seed Pudding with Coconut Milk Quinoa Bowl with Vegetables Stuffed Bell Peppers with Meat Dried Mango Make extra quinoa for lunch

Friday Green Smoothie with Avocado AIP Tacos with Lettuce Wraps Grilled Chicken with Broccoli Plantain Chips with Salsa Marinate chicken for grilling

Saturday Banana Pancakes with Maple Syrup Chicken Soup Roasted Vegetables Cucumber Slices with Hummus Prepare soup in bulk for meals

Sunday Omelette with Spinach Salad with Lemon Dressing Spaghetti Squash with Sauce Trail Mix with Nuts Cook extra spaghetti squash

Digital Meal Planning Apps

Consider using meal planning apps like Mealime or Plan to Eat. These tools allow you to collect recipes, create grocery lists, and personalize your meal plans effortlessly. They can also provide ideas and help you track what you've enjoyed eating.

Strategies for Batch Cooking and Meal Prep

Batch cooking and meal prep are game-changers for anyone following the AIP Diet. By preparing large quantities of food at once, you may save time, decrease stress, and ensure that you always have healthy meals ready to go.

Plan Your Batch Cooking Sessions

Choose one or two days a week for batch cooking. Sundays are a popular choice, as they allow you to plan meals for the week ahead. However, feel free to pick a day that suits your schedule best.

Cook in Batches

Cook greater servings of staples including grains, meats, and veggies. For example:

Roast a tray of different vegetables to enjoy throughout the week.

Make a large pot of bone broth that can be used in soups or as a foundation for sauces.

Grill or bake various parts of chicken, which can be sliced for salads or wraps.

Use Freezer-Friendly Recipes

Make dishes that store well, such as stews, soups, and casseroles. Portion them into containers and label them with the contents and date. This can help you prevent food waste and give you quick supper options on busy days.

Organize Your Refrigerator and Freezer

Keep your prepped meals organized by labeling containers and keeping them in a readily accessible manner. Create a special shelf for prepped meals so you can quickly find what you need.

Stay Flexible

Life can be unpredictable, so allow for flexibility in your food planning. Having a few basic backup meals on hand, such as frozen veggies or pre-cooked proteins, might help you stay on track even when your plans change.

Cooking Techniques for AIP

Cooking procedures play a key impact in the quality and nutritional worth of your meals. The methods you choose can enhance the flavors and preserve the nutrients of the ingredients you're utilizing.

Essential Kitchen Tools and Equipment

Equipping your kitchen with the correct tools can make a major impact in your cooking experience. Here's a list of necessary kitchen gadgets that can help you survive on the AIP Diet:

Sharp Knives

Invest in a nice set of knives for chopping, slicing, and dicing. A sharp chef's knife and a paring knife can cover most of your cutting needs.

Cutting Boards

Use separate chopping boards for vegetables and proteins to avoid cross-contamination. Consider having both wood and plastic boards; wooden boards are wonderful for veggies, while plastic is easy to disinfect for proteins.

Food Processor

A food processor can save you time when cooking meals. Use it for cutting vegetables, producing purees, or creating nut butters (if tolerated).

Blender

A high-quality blender is vital for creating smoothies, soups, and sauces. Look for one with a robust motor to handle frozen fruits and fibrous veggies.

Slow Cooker or Instant Pot

These appliances are wonderful for meal prep. Use a slow cooker for stews, soups, and roasts that may cook throughout the day. The Instant

Pot gives the same benefits but with the extra bonus of speed.

Baking Sheets and Casserole Dishes

Invest in good-quality baking sheets and casserole dishes for roasting veggies, baking meats, and producing one-pan dinners.

Glass Storage Containers

Use glass containers for storing prepped meals in the refrigerator or freezer. They are resilient, easy to clean, and won't leach chemicals into your food.

Spiralizer

A spiralizer is great for generating vegetable noodles, such as zucchini or sweet potato noodles. This might be a fun way to integrate extra vegetables into your meals.

Cooking Methods that Preserve Nutrients

The manner you cook your food can alter its nutritional worth. Here are some AIP-friendly cooking methods that help preserve nutrients:

Steaming

Steaming veggies retains more vitamins and minerals than boiling. Use a steamer basket over a pot of boiling water or invest in a dedicated steamer.

Sautéing

Sautéing veggies in a modest amount of healthy oil, like olive or avocado oil, allows them to keep their nutrients while improving their flavors. Be careful not to overcook; aim for tender-crisp textures.

Roasting

Roasting brings out the inherent sweetness of vegetables and enriches their flavors. Use high heat (about 400-425°F) for optimal results. Toss vegetables with oil and herbs before putting them on a baking sheet.

Slow Cooking

Slow cooking meats and stews at low temperatures helps tastes to melt together while retaining moisture and nutrients. This procedure is particularly good for harder cuts of meat.

Fermenting

Fermenting foods like vegetables increases their nutritional value and enhances gut health. Consider creating your own sauerkraut or pickles using a simple brine.

Blanching

Quickly blanching vegetables in boiling water and then plunging them into freezing water maintains their color, texture, and nutrition. This method is useful for prepping vegetables for freezing.

Meal planning and preparation are key components of your journey on the AIP Diet. By making a weekly meal plan, employing batch cooking procedures, and mastering cooking techniques that maintain nutrients, you'll set yourself up for success.

Chapter 5: Simple AIP Recipes

Embarking on the Autoimmune Protocol (AIP) diet doesn't mean abandoning flavor or innovation in the kitchen. In fact, it opens up a universe of culinary possibilities that celebrate wholesome products while feeding your body. This chapter is filled with simple, delicious AIP dishes across all meals—breakfast, lunch, supper, snacks, and desserts. Whether you're an expert cook or just starting, these recipes are designed to be approachable and gratifying, helping you embrace your AIP journey with joy and simplicity.

Breakfast Ideas

Starting your day with a good breakfast is vital, especially when following the AIP diet. Breakfast sets the tone for your day, delivering energy and nutrients that feed your body. Here are some great breakfast options that are both healthy and easy to prepare.

1. AIP Smoothie Bowl

Ingredients:

1 cup spinach (fresh or frozen)

1 banana

1/2 cup coconut milk (canned or carton)

1 tbsp chia seeds

1/2 teaspoon vanilla extract

Toppings: sliced kiwi, coconut flakes, and pumpkin seeds

Instructions:

In a blender, add spinach, banana, coconut milk, chia seeds, and vanilla extract. Blend until smooth.

Pour the smoothie into a bowl and top with sliced kiwi, coconut flakes, and pumpkin seeds.

Enjoy immediately as a refreshing and nutrient-packed breakfast!

2. Sweet Potato Hash

Ingredients:

2 medium sweet potatoes, diced

1 bell pepper, diced

1 small onion, chopped

2 tablespoons olive oil

Salt and pepper to taste

Fresh herbs (parsley or cilantro) for garnish

Instructions:

In a large skillet, heat olive oil over medium heat. Add the sweet potatoes and simmer for about 10 minutes, stirring periodically, until they begin to soften.

Add the bell pepper and onion to the skillet. Season with salt and pepper. Cook for another 5-7 minutes until the vegetables are soft and caramelized.

Garnish with fresh herbs before serving. This vibrant meal is a terrific way to start your day with fiber and minerals.

3. Banana Pancakes

Ingredients:

2 ripe bananas

2 eggs (or 1/4 cup applesauce for egg-free option)

1/2 teaspoon cinnamon

1 tablespoon coconut oil for cooking

Instructions:

In a bowl, mash the bananas until smooth. Add eggs (or applesauce) and cinnamon, mixing well.

Heat coconut oil in a skillet over medium heat. Pour little amounts of batter onto the skillet to produce pancakes.

Cook for roughly 2-3 minutes on each side until golden brown. Serve warm with fresh fruit or a dollop of maple syrup.

Lunch Recipes

A healthy lunch is vital for maintaining energy levels throughout the day. Here are some simple and excellent AIP lunch recipes that will keep you full and focused.

4. Colorful AIP Salad

Ingredients:

2 cups mixed leafy greens (spinach, arugula, or romaine)

1/2 cucumber, sliced

1/2 cup cherry tomatoes, halved

1/4 avocado, diced

1/4 cup shredded carrots

Dressing: 2 tablespoons olive oil, 1 tablespoon apple cider vinegar, salt, and pepper to taste

Instructions:

In a large bowl, add the leafy greens, cucumber, cherry tomatoes, avocado, and carrots.

In a small bowl, whisk together olive oil, apple cider vinegar, salt, and pepper. Drizzle the dressing over the salad and toss to mix.

Enjoy this fresh, colorful salad that's rich of vitamins and healthy fats.

5. AIP Chicken Soup

Ingredients:

1 pound boneless, skinless chicken thighs

4 cups chicken broth (homemade or store-bought, verify for AIP compliance)

2 carrots, sliced

2 celery stalks, cut

1 onion, diced

2 cloves garlic, minced

1 teaspoon dried thyme

Salt and pepper to taste

Instructions:

In a big pot, heat a splash of olive oil over medium heat. Add onions and garlic, sautéing until fragrant.

Add chicken thighs, broth, carrots, celery, thyme, salt, and pepper. Bring to a boil, then reduce heat and let simmer for about 25 minutes.

Once the chicken is cooked, shred it with two forks and return it to the pot. Adjust seasoning as needed. Serve warm and comforting!

6. Turkey Lettuce Wraps

Ingredients:

1 pound ground turkey

1 tbsp coconut aminos

1 tablespoon olive oil

1 bell pepper, diced

1 small onion, chopped

Lettuce leaves (romaine or butter lettuce) for wrapping

Instructions:

In a skillet, heat olive oil over medium heat. Add onions and bell peppers, simmering until softened.

Add ground turkey and coconut aminos, cooking until the turkey is fully cooked and browned. Season with salt and pepper.

Serve the turkey mixture in lettuce leaves, adding toppings such sliced cucumbers or avocado if preferred.

Dinner Dishes

Dinner is the perfect occasion to produce warm, cozy dishes that are both nutritional and fulfilling. Here are some great AIP-friendly dinner recipes that showcase meats, fish, and colorful greens.

7. Herb-Crusted Baked Salmon

Ingredients:

2 salmon fillets

2 tablespoons olive oil

1 tablespoon lemon juice

1 tablespoon fresh dill, chopped

Salt and pepper to taste

Instructions:

Preheat the oven to 375°F (190°C). Line a baking sheet with parchment paper.

In a bowl, mix olive oil, lemon juice, dill, salt, and pepper. Brush the mixture over the salmon fillets.

Place the fillets on the prepared baking sheet and bake for 15-20 minutes or until cooked through and flaky. Serve with steamed vegetables for a complete dinner.

8. Stuffed Bell Peppers

Ingredients:

4 bell peppers (any color)

1 pound ground beef or turkey

1 cup cooked cauliflower rice

1 teaspoon Italian seasoning

Salt and pepper to taste

Instructions:

Preheat the oven to 375°F (190°C). Cut the tops off the bell peppers and remove the seeds.

In a skillet, sauté the ground meat over medium heat until browned. Stir in cauliflower rice, Italian seasoning, salt, and pepper.

Stuff the bell peppers with the meat mixture and set them upright in a baking tray. Add a splash of water to the bottom of the dish and cover with foil.

Bake for 30-35 minutes, removing the foil for the last 10 minutes. Enjoy these colorful and hearty stuffed peppers!

9. Zucchini Noodles with Meat Sauce

Ingredients:

2 medium zucchinis, spiralized

1 pound ground meat (beef, turkey, or pork)

1 can (14 oz) crushed tomatoes (confirm for AIP compliance)

1 teaspoon dried basil

Salt and pepper to taste

2 tablespoons olive oil

Instructions:

In a large skillet, heat olive oil over medium heat. Add ground meat and heat until browned.

Stir in crushed tomatoes, basil, salt, and pepper. Let the sauce boil for 10-15 minutes.

In another pan, softly sauté the zucchini noodles until just tender. Serve the meat sauce over the noodles for a warm, noodle-free pasta dish.

Snacks and Desserts

Satisfying your appetites with healthy snacks and treats is crucial to keeping balance on the AIP diet. Here are some great options that will keep you satisfied between meals.

10. AIP Trail Mix

Ingredients:

1/2 cup coconut flakes (unsweetened)

1/4 cup pumpkin seeds

1/4 cup dried cranberries (unsweetened)

1/4 cup sunflower seeds

Instructions:

In a mixing bowl, add coconut flakes, pumpkin seeds, dried cranberries, and sunflower seeds.

Store in an airtight container for a quick, on-the-go snack that's filled with healthy fats and fiber.

11. Carrot Sticks with AIP Hummus

Ingredients for Hummus:

1 can (15 oz) chickpeas (optional; for rigorous AIP, substitute with cauliflower)

1 cup cooked cauliflower florets

1/4 cup tahini

2 tablespoons olive oil

Juice of 1 lemon

Salt to taste

Instructions:

In a blender or food processor, combine chickpeas (or cauliflower), tahini, olive oil, lemon juice, and salt. Blend until smooth, adding a little water if necessary to obtain the desired consistency.

Serve with carrot sticks for a crunchy, delicious snack.

12. AIP Chocolate Avocado Mousse

Ingredients:

1 ripe avocado

1/4 cup cocoa powder (unsweetened)

1/4 cup maple syrup

1 teaspoon vanilla extract

Pinch of salt

Instructions:

In a food processor, blend avocado, cocoa powder, maple syrup, vanilla extract, and salt. Blend till creamy and smooth.

Spoon the mousse into serving dishes and chill for 30 minutes before enjoying this rich and luscious dessert.

These AIP recipes indicate that healthy eating can be both simple and enjoyable. From vivid breakfast bowls to hefty dinners and comforting snacks, there's something for everyone in this collection. As you explore these recipes, feel free to get creative by mixing and matching ingredients to suit your preferences. The AIP journey is about sustaining your body while enjoying the act of preparing and sharing meals with loved ones. Enjoy every bite as you embrace a healthier lifestyle!

Chapter 6: Overcoming Challenges on AIP

Transitioning to the Autoimmune Protocol (AIP) diet can be a transformative path toward better health, but it's not without its hurdles. From cravings for familiar foods to navigating social situations and managing money restraints, many people find obstacles when adopting this lifestyle. This chapter will discuss major issues related with AIP and suggest practical solutions to overcome them. Additionally, we will address the need of emotional and psychological support along your AIP journey, helping you create resilience and sustain drive.

Common Challenges and Solutions

Embarking on the AIP diet can feel daunting at times, especially when cravings strike, or social occasions arise. Here, we'll discuss some of the most prevalent challenges and practical solutions to help you stay on track.

1. Dealing with Cravings and Social Situations

Understanding Cravings

Cravings are a natural component of any dietary adjustment, especially when eliminating foods that may have been staples in your former diet. On AIP, common cravings could include grains, dairy, and sweet foods. Recognizing that cravings frequently come from emotional or physical stimuli might help you negotiate them more effectively.

Solutions:

Healthy Substitutes: Instead of grabbing for a sugary snack or a bowl of spaghetti, have a list of AIP-friendly alternatives handy. For example, if you need something sweet, try creating AIP chocolate avocado mousse or fruit-based desserts. When wanting comfort foods like pasta, spiralized zucchini or sweet potatoes might be a pleasant option.

Mindful Eating: Practice mindful eating practices to help manage urges. When you notice a craving, halt and take a moment to examine your appetite. Are you actually hungry, or are you desiring for emotional reasons? Engage in a brief meditation or deep breathing practice to check in with your body.

Plan Ahead for Social circumstances: Social events can pose a difficulty when following AIP, but with enough planning, you can manage these circumstances comfortably. Consider the following strategies:

Bring Your Own Dish: Offer to bring a dish that you can enjoy and share with others. This way, you can assure that there's something AIP-friendly at the event.

Communicate Your Needs: Don't hesitate to inform your friends or family about your dietary limitations. Most folks would appreciate your honesty and may even offer to cook something AIP-friendly.

attention on Socializing, Not Food: Shift your attention during social occasions from food to connection. Engage in conversations and activities that don't concentrate around eating, such as playing games, dancing, or appreciating nature.

2. Addressing Budget Constraints

Switching to AIP can sometimes feel financially overwhelming, especially with the emphasis on high-quality, complete foods. However, it's possible to manage your finances properly while keeping an AIP lifestyle.

Solutions:

Meal organizing & Bulk Cooking: Save money by organizing your meals for the week. Create a shopping list based on your food plan to avoid impulse purchases. Batch cooking can also help you prepare numerous meals at once, cutting cooking time and costs.

Shop Seasonal and Local: Seasonal produce is often more inexpensive and fresher than out-of-season selections. Visit local farmers' markets or community-supported agriculture (CSA) programs for fresh, in-season fruits and vegetables.

Buy in Bulk: Stock up on AIP-friendly pantry basics like coconut flour, olive oil, and herbs by purchasing them in bulk. Many stores provide discounts for buying greater quantities, which might save you money in the long term.

Prioritize Quality Over Quantity: Focus on buying high-quality meats and veggies, but consider reducing portion sizes to stretch your money further. For example, instead of using a full chicken for a meal, you can roast a smaller bird and use the leftovers in several recipes during the week.

Emotional and Psychological Support

Embarking on an AIP journey isn't only about nutritional changes; it also entails emotional and psychological adaptations. Developing a solid support system and integrating self-care routines will help you manage these changes more successfully.

1. Mindfulness and Self-Care Practices

The Role of Mindfulness

Mindfulness methods, including as meditation, yoga, and deep breathing, can dramatically enhance your experience on AIP. These activities help you stay grounded and present, enabling you to better control cravings and emotional triggers.

Self-Care Practices:

Everyday Meditation: Incorporate a short meditation practice into your everyday routine. Even five minutes of focused breathing can help calm your thoughts and minimize anxiety associated to dietary changes.

Journaling: Keep a journal to chart your AIP journey, including your feelings, struggles, and accomplishments. Writing can be a therapeutic outlet, letting you process your experiences and reflect on your progress.

Gentle Movement: Engage in gentle types of exercise that you love, such as walking, yoga, or swimming. Movement can help release endorphins, increase your mood, and decrease stress.

Gratitude Practice: Cultivating gratitude might boost your emotional resilience. Each day, take a time to focus on three things you are grateful for, whether they pertain to your health, relationships, or personal achievements.

2. Building a Support System

Having a supportive network is vital when negotiating the obstacles of the AIP diet. Connecting with individuals who share similar experiences can bring encouragement, motivation, and useful insights.

Building Your Support System:

Online Communities: Join AIP-focused online communities, forums, or social media groups. These areas give opportunities to discuss your journey, seek guidance, and connect with others who understand the issues you face.

Local Support Groups: If possible, seek out local support groups for persons following AIP or dealing with autoimmune disorders. Meeting in person can develop stronger ties and provide a sense of belonging.

Involve Friends and Family: Educate your friends and family about the AIP diet and its benefits. Encourage them to help you by learning more about your dietary preferences and maybe joining you in trying new meals.

Seek Professional Guidance: Consider working with a licensed dietitian or nutritionist who specializes in the AIP diet. They can provide personalized coaching, help you build food plans, and offer essential insights to support your journey.

Overcoming the challenges of the AIP diet demands commitment, inventiveness, and a willingness to adapt. By knowing frequent barriers and implementing practical methods, you may manage your AIP journey with confidence and perseverance. Remember to prioritize self-care and seek help from others, allowing yourself the grace to learn and grow along the way. Your commitment to this lifestyle can lead to remarkable health gains, and with patience and perseverance, you will find the joys of nourishing your body and spirit through AIP.

Chapter 7: Success Stories and Testimonials

The Autoimmune Protocol (AIP) diet has transformed countless lives, bringing hope and healing to people facing autoimmune illnesses and chronic inflammation. While scientific studies and theoretical frameworks provide vital insights into the AIP diet's mechanics, nothing resonates quite like personal stories of triumph. In this chapter, we will analyze real-life transformations from individuals who have embraced the AIP lifestyle. Through their testimonials, we will explore the struggles they faced, the lessons they learned, and the inspirational improvements that followed.

Real-Life Transformations

Every AIP journey is unique, shaped by particular circumstances and health concerns. The following anecdotes show the different experiences of persons who have adopted the AIP diet, bringing light on their problems, achievements, and novel perspectives on health and wellness.

1. Emily's Journey: From Chronic Fatigue to Vibrant Health

Background:

Emily, a 32-year-old graphic designer, had been battling with persistent exhaustion and joint discomfort for several years. Diagnosed with Hashimoto's thyroiditis, she often found herself weary and unable to keep up with her busy career and social life. After multiple doctor visits and drugs that failed to bring relief, Emily discovered the AIP diet through an online support group.

The Turning Point:

Emily chose to commit entirely to the AIP lifestyle, considering it as her final option for regaining her health. She started by reviewing her current diet and eliminating inflammatory foods, including wheat, dairy, and processed sugars. Initially, the shift was tough; Emily experienced intense cravings and struggled to adapt to the new culinary techniques required for AIP.

The Transformation:

Within a few weeks, Emily saw considerable improvements. Her energy levels began to climb, and the joint discomfort that had tormented her for years started to subside. Inspired by these improvements, she took the time to learn about meal planning and preparation, creating delicious AIP-friendly meals that brought joy back into her kitchen.

"I had no idea food could have such a profound impact on how I felt," Emily shared. "It was empowering to see the connection between what I was eating and how my body responded. I started feeling like my old self again."

Lessons Learned:

Emily learned the significance of patience and self-compassion during her path. While she encountered setbacks, she got a deeper awareness of her body and the triggers that produced her symptoms. Emily now campaigns for AIP within her community, sharing her story to urge others to take ownership of their health.

2.   Jason's Transformation: Overcoming Inflammatory Bowel Disease

Background:

Jason, a 45-year-old father of two, experienced the severe affects of inflammatory bowel disease (IBD) for over a decade. Frequent flare-ups left him unable to enjoy family excursions and engage in activities he liked. After attending a health lecture, Jason learnt about the AIP diet and its potential benefits for those with autoimmune diseases.

The Turning Point:

Determined to take control of his health, Jason went on the AIP adventure. He began by painstakingly removing trigger items and integrating nutrient-dense options into his diet. Initially, the lifestyle shift was intimidating, but he found solace in the support of internet networks and local AIP meet-ups.

The Transformation:

As weeks evolved into months, Jason experienced a stunning metamorphosis. His symptoms began to lessen, allowing him to enjoy family activities without worry of abrupt flare-ups. "For the first time in years, I felt free," Jason remarked. "I could play with my kids without worrying about my stomach. I even went on a camping vacation, something I hadn't done in forever."

Lessons Learned:

Jason's adventure taught him the value of community and support. He connected with people suffering similar issues, which gave him both encouragement and accountability. Additionally, Jason realized the value of self-care and stress management, including mindfulness practices into his routine to promote his general well-being.

3. Sarah's Experience: Healing Through Mindful Eating

Background:

Sarah, a 29-year-old yoga instructor, had been diagnosed with lupus, which left her feeling overwhelmed and nervous about her health. Despite being active and health-conscious, she struggled with constant inflammation, exhaustion, and joint pain. After investigating natural alternatives to healing, Sarah landed discovered the AIP diet.

The Turning Point:

Curious about the possible benefits, Sarah decided to try with AIP. She began by maintaining a food journal to monitor her meals and symptoms. This practice allowed her to identify triggers and trends in her diet that contributed to her inflammation.

The Transformation:

As she embraced the AIP lifestyle, Sarah found herself not only recuperating physically but also building a deeper connection to her body. "Eating became a mindful practice for me," she stated. "I learned to appreciate every bite and understand how food nourished me. It was like a type of self-love."

Sarah noted considerable increases in her energy levels and reduced joint pain. Her experience with AIP also inspired her to investigate other forms of self-care, like meditation and yoga, which further boosted her well-being.

Lessons Learned:

Through her experience, Sarah learned the significance of listening to her body and honoring its demands. She learned that healing is a holistic process, embracing not just food modifications but also emotional and spiritual well-being. Sarah now shares her story on social media, motivating others to approach their health journeys with mindfulness and intention.

4. *Mark's Success: A Journey of Resilience*

Background:

Mark, a 50-year-old software developer, has been diagnosed with multiple sclerosis (MS). Faced with debilitating symptoms that disrupted his daily existence, he felt a sense of helplessness. After investigating dietary therapies, he decided to give the AIP diet a try.

The Turning Point:

Mark's commitment to AIP was fuelled by a desire to restore his life. He faced hurdles as he avoided packaged foods and learnt to cook with novel items. However, he stayed dedicated to his aim of lowering inflammation and improving his health.

The Transformation:

Over time, Mark noticed a dramatic reduction in symptoms, allowing him to engage in things he had enjoyed, like hiking and playing guitar. "I never thought I could feel this good again," Mark shared. "The AIP diet has given me my life back."

Mark's journey was not without obstacles, but he learnt the power of tenacity and flexibility. He found that setbacks were a natural part of the healing process and that tenacity was crucial to overcoming challenges.

Lessons Learned:

Mark underlined the significance of recognizing tiny accomplishments along the road. He learnt to acknowledge his progress, no matter how modest, and to seek help from friends and family when needed. Mark now advises individuals with autoimmune disorders to investigate dietary modifications as a method of empowerment.

Inspirational Stories and Lessons Learned

The anecdotes provided in this chapter highlight the different experiences of individuals who have achieved success with the AIP diet. Each journey is unique, yet common themes emerge:

Empowerment via Knowledge: Individuals who adopted AIP typically described feeling empowered by the knowledge they received about their bodies and the impact of food on their health.

Community Support: Many success stories highlight the benefits of interacting with people on similar journeys. Whether through online forums, local meet-ups, or supportive friends and family, community plays a critical part in preserving motivation and responsibility.

Mindful Practices: The practice of mindfulness—whether through mindful eating, meditation, or self-reflection—has emerged as a powerful tool for negotiating the emotional and psychological elements of dietary changes.

Resilience and Adaptability: The route toward health is often characterized with ups and downs. Those that succeed learn to be resilient and adaptive, realizing that failures are a natural part of the process.

As you reflect on these inspiring experiences, realize that your path with the AIP diet is uniquely yours. While problems may arise, the transformations and accomplishments that others have experienced can serve as strong motivation. Embrace the process of healing, and take comfort in knowing that you are not alone on this road. The AIP diet can be a route toward improved health, vitality, and empowerment, bringing hope and healing for anyone willing to explore its potential. Let these success stories motivate you to take the next step toward your own transformation.

Chapter 8: Maintaining Your Health Beyond AIP

Embarking on the Autoimmune Protocol (AIP) diet can be a transforming experience, leading to major gains in health, vigor, and overall well-being. As you traverse the road of healing and reclaiming your life, it's vital to think about what happens next. How can you preserve the beneficial adjustments you've made while continuing to support your body in the long term? This chapter will walk you through the critical processes for safely reintroduction foods, monitoring your body's reactions, and building sustainable lifestyle practices that compliment your AIP journey.

Reintroducing Foods Safely

One of the most essential aspects of the AIP journey is the reintroduction of meals after finishing the elimination phase. This approach can be both thrilling and intimidating, as it offers the opportunity of enjoying a greater choice of meals while ensuring you remain attentive of how your body responds.

Guidelines for Food Reintroduction

Start Slowly: Begin by reintroducing one food at a time. This allows you to correctly assess your body's reaction to each individual item without the complexity of several variables. Ideally, wait at least three to five days between introducing new foods to give your body time to acclimate.

Choose Your Foods Wisely: Select foods that are known to be less inflammatory or widely tolerated by others who have followed AIP. For instance, after the initial period, consider reintroducing foods like sweet potatoes, non-gluten grains (such as quinoa or millet), or some herbs and spices.

Keep a Food Journal: Document your reintroductions in a food journal. Record what you consume, the quantity, and any symptoms or reactions you have. This record will be essential for identifying potential dietary triggers and understanding your body's unique responses.

Pay Attention to Symptoms: After introducing a new food, examine your body for any unfavorable reactions. Common signs to check for include digestive troubles (bloating, gas, diarrhea), skin reactions (rashes, hives), joint discomfort, weariness, or mental changes. If you experience any serious symptoms, consider removing the food and waiting a week before trying again.

Be Patient: Allow yourself grace during this process. Your body may take time to adjust, and some meals may not be good for you at this period. Remember that the goal is to learn what works for you and to prioritize your health and well-being.

Monitoring Reactions and Symptoms

Understanding how your body responds to reintroduced meals is vital for sustaining your health post-AIP. As you reintroduce foods, here are some strategies for properly monitoring reactions and symptoms:

Stay Aware of Subtle Changes: Sometimes, reactions might be subtle and may not occur immediately. Be careful for delayed responses that could occur hours or even days after consuming a specific item.

Seek Professional Guidance: If you are uncertain about your reactions or need assistance with the reintroduction process, consider speaking with a healthcare professional, such as a registered dietitian who specializes in autoimmune diseases. They can provide specialized guidance and support tailored to your needs.

Stay Open-Minded: Reintroducing foods is a personal experience, and what works for one person may not work for another. Approach the process with curiosity and an open mind, allowing yourself the ability to adjust and discover what feels best for your body.

Long-Term Lifestyle Strategies

As you advance beyond the AIP diet, it's crucial to build long-term lifestyle habits that support sustainable health and well-being. Here are some crucial topics to focus on when you adopt AIP into a healthy lifestyle:

Integrating AIP into a Balanced Lifestyle

Maintain Mindful Eating Habits: Continue to prioritize complete, nutrient-dense foods while remaining flexible in your approach. Mindful eating enables you to savor your meals, appreciate the flavors, and identify when you are satisfied. This practice creates a healthy relationship with food and helps you remain in tune with your body's needs.

Be Selective with Food Choices: While the AIP diet provides a solid basis, you don't have to rigidly adhere to it forever. Allow yourself to eat a range of foods, including some of your favorites, in moderation. Focus on quality over quantity, choosing organic and minimally processed meals whenever possible.

Stay Informed: Keep learning about diet and health. The science of nutrition is ever-evolving, and staying educated about new studies, recipes, and recommendations can help you adapt your approach to food and health over time.

Cultivate Community: Maintain connections with those who understand your experience. Whether through local support groups, online forums, or social media communities, having a network of like-minded folks can provide encouragement, inspiration, and accountability as you navigate your health path.

Other Complementary Healing Practices

Prioritize Exercise: Regular physical activity is a cornerstone of overall health. Find a workout program that you enjoy, whether it's yoga, walking, swimming, or strength training. Aim for at least 150 minutes of moderate activity each week, embracing activities that boost both physical and mental well-being.

Focus on Sleep: Quality sleep is crucial for recovery and overall health. Establish a consistent sleep schedule, build a calm nighttime routine, and ensure your sleep environment is favorable to peaceful sleep. Consider strategies such as minimizing screen time before bed, reducing coffee intake in the afternoon, and creating a comfortable sleeping place.

Incorporate Stress Management: Chronic stress can increase autoimmune symptoms and delay healing. Explore numerous stress management approaches such as mindfulness meditation, deep breathing exercises, journaling, or spending time in nature. Find what works best for you and make it a priority in your daily routine.

Consider Integrative Therapies: Complementary therapies, such as acupuncture, chiropractic care, or massage therapy, can support your healing process. These techniques may help ease symptoms, reduce stress, and enhance general well-being. Consult with healthcare professionals to investigate which therapies might be good for you.

Stay Hydrated: Proper hydration is vital for sustaining good health. Drink plenty of water throughout the day and consider incorporating herbal teas or infused water for extra flavor and nutrition. Staying hydrated improves digestion, skin health, and overall bodily processes.

Continue Learning About Your Body: As you venture beyond AIP, remain curious about your body's unique sensitivities to different meals, activities, and situations. By actively listening to your body, you'll be better equipped to make informed decisions that correspond with your health goals.

Embracing a New Chapter

As you end your AIP journey and transition into a new chapter of health and wellness, remember that the process is continuous. Maintaining your health beyond AIP is about finding balance, recognizing your body's cues, and embracing a lifestyle that fosters vitality and joy.

The tools and insights you've gained along this trip can serve as a blueprint for continued success. Embrace the changes you've made, and allow them to enable you to live a meaningful, vibrant life. Whether you want to adhere to the AIP principles, integrate new foods, or explore supplementary methods, the goal is to prioritize your well-being.

Remember, this trip is uniquely yours. Celebrate your progress, acknowledge your problems, and continue to seek joy in the process of healing. With each step, you are crafting a life that values your health, embraces your individuality, and supports your brilliant future. The road may be ongoing, but you now possess the tools, knowledge, and resilience to thrive.

Conclusion: Embracing a Life of Health and Balance

As you stand at the completion of this research into the Autoimmune Protocol (AIP), it's necessary to take a minute to think on the journey you've done and the life changes that await you. This conclusion is not just an end; it is a celebration of your commitment to health, a roadmap for your ongoing journey, and an encouragement to embrace a future filled with balance, vitality, and self-discovery.

The Commitment to Healing

The route to wellness is rarely a straight line. It's often a meandering route filled with ups and downs, moments of victory, and difficulties that test your determination. Committing to the AIP is a brave step toward repairing your body from the inside out, and it is a tribute to your desire for a healthier, more vibrant life. As you embark on this lifestyle, remember that consistency is vital. Each meal you prepare, each thoughtful decision you make, and each supportive community connection you develop plays a crucial impact in your recovery path.

Embracing Change

One of the most crucial lessons learnt via the AIP experience is the power of adaptation. You may have discovered new foods, flavors, and techniques that have transformed how you perceive nutrition. You may have created new habits that foster mindful eating and a better connection to your body. Embracing these adjustments can be a tremendous catalyst for transformation, not only in your physical health but in every part of your life.

The Importance of Mindset

Your mindset is a critical component of your health journey. By choosing to view problems as opportunities for progress, you cultivate resilience. There will be days when sticking to the AIP feels daunting, and desires for familiar foods may entice you. In these moments, it's crucial to remind yourself of your goals, the benefits you've already experienced, and the empowerment that comes from making conscious choices for your well-being.

Stay curious and open to learning during this process. Nutrition research is ever-evolving, and as you find what works for your body, remain flexible in your approach. Seek out new recipes, explore different cooking techniques, and heed to your body's messages. This journey is not simply about keeping to a rigid set of principles; it's about establishing a nourishing relationship with food and yourself.

The Power of Community

The contacts you build within the AIP community can serve as a tremendous source of support. As you travel this journey, surround yourself with those that elevate and support you. Share your triumphs, no matter how modest, and lean on others during hard times. The sensation of belonging can be tremendously motivating and may change what may feel like an onerous trip into a shared experience filled with friendship.

Consider joining in local meetups, communicating with online forums, or simply reaching out to fellow AIP aficionados. Together, you may swap recipes, share stories, and celebrate triumphs, creating a network of support that encourages your commitment to recovering.

Mindfulness and Self-Discovery

Throughout your trip, practicing mindfulness will help you remain grounded and centered. Take the time to check in with yourself periodically. How does your body feel? What feelings arise when you think of food and nourishment? Mindfulness can bring vital insights that lead to self-discovery and a greater knowledge of your relationship with food.

As you embrace the AIP lifestyle, consider adopting extra self-care behaviors that enhance general well-being. Engage in hobbies that bring you delight, such as yoga, meditation, or simply spending time in nature. Prioritize adequate sleep and physical activity, realizing that these factors are crucial to overall health. By supporting your mind, body, and spirit, you establish the framework for sustained recovery and growth.

Celebrating Your Journey

Celebrate the progress you've achieved, whether great and small. Whether you've discovered a new favorite recipe, noticed a reduction in symptoms, or simply learnt to relish each bite, every step forward is worth appreciating.

Document your journey through journaling or photography, documenting the moments of delight and accomplishment. These reflections can serve as powerful reminders of your tenacity and dedication when situations get tough.

A Future of Balance and Well-Being

As you move forward, keep your sights set on the horizon of what is possible. The AIP diet is not simply a temporary remedy; it is a pathway to a life of balance, vigor, and well-being. The insights learnt during this journey might extend beyond eating, informing your total approach to health and life.

Integrate what you've learned into your daily routine, seeking to maintain a diet rich in whole, nutrient-dense foods even beyond the organized phases of the AIP. Continue to listen to your body, honoring its demands and modifying your lifestyle as appropriate. Recognize that health is not only the absence of disease; it is the presence of life and joy.

Final Thoughts

In closing, the Autoimmune Protocol is more than a nutritional framework; it is a lifestyle choice built in self-compassion and empowerment. It is about reclaiming your health, cultivating a profound relationship with your body, and embracing the journey of self-discovery.

Allow this moment to be the beginning of a revolutionary chapter in your life. Embrace the unknown, cherish the journey, and remain devoted to healing. As you pursue this path, may you find strength in your decisions, joy in your discoveries, and peace in your body and mind.

Remember, you are not alone on this path. A community of persons, resources, and information stands ready to support you every step of the way. Together, you can develop a new narrative—one of health, balance, and empowerment—celebrating the power of food, connection, and self-care.

Thank you for allowing this examination of the AIP to occur in your life. Here's to a future filled with bright health, joy, and the ongoing adventure of self-discovery!

The end